PREHENSION ASSESSMENT

Prosthetic Therapy for the Upper-Limb Child Amputee

David Krebs, Editor

PREHENSION ASSESSMENT

Prosthetic Therapy for the Upper-Limb Child Amputee

David Krebs, Editor

SLACK Incorporated, 6900 Grove Road , Thorofare, New Jersey 08086

The editor and publisher acknowledge sincere appreciation for photographs, including the photograph used on the cover, supplied by Mr. T. Wally Williams, III of the Liberty Mutual Research Center.

Printed in the United States of America

Library of Congress Catalog Card Number: 87-61367

ISBN: 1-55642-021-8

Published by: SLACK Incorporated
                     6900 Grove Road
                     Thorofare, NJ 08086

Last digit is print number: 10 9 8 7 6 5 4 3 2 1

CONTENTS

LIST OF PARTICIPANTS

Diane Atkins, OT
Houston Center for Amputee Services
The Institute for Rehabiliation and Research
1333 Moursund
Houston, TX 77030

Felice Celikyol, OT
Kessler Institute for Rehabilitation
1199 Pleasant Valley Way
West Orange, NJ 07052

Susan D. Clarke, OT
Child Amputee Prosthetics Project
University of California
1000 Veteran Avenue
Los Angeles, CA 90024

Patricia C. Cope, OT
Juvenile Amputee Clinic
Handicapped Children's Services
19th and Massachusetts Avenues, S.E.
Washington, DC 20003

Joan Edelstein, PT
New York University
Post-Graduate Medical School
317 East 34th Street
New York, NY 10016

Ellen B. Hamburg, OT
Kernan Hospital Amputee and Prosthetic Clinic
2200 North Forest Park Avenue
Baltimore, MD 21207

Donabelle Hansen, PT
Shriners Hospitals for Crippled Children
Twin Cities Unit
2025 East River Road
Minneapolis, MN 55414

Sheila Hubbard, PT, OT
Ontario Crippled Children's Centre
Paediatric Rehabilitation Centre
350 Rumsey Road
Toronto, Ontario
Canada M4G-IR8

David E. Krebs, PT
New York University
Post-Graduate Medical School
317 East 34th Street
New York, NY 10016

Anne M. Laband, OT
Kernan Hospital Amputee and Prosthetic Clinic
2200 North Forest Park Avenue
Baltimore, MD 21207

William Neill, PT
Kernan Hospital Amputee and Prosthetic Clinic
2200 North Forest Park Avenue
Baltimore, MD 21207

Joanna Patton, OT
UCLA Child Amputee Project
Rehabilitation Center
Room 25-26
1000 Veteran Avenue
Los Angeles, CA 90024

Elizabeth Sanderson, OT
Fredericton Myoelectric Prosthetics Clinic
Forest Hill Rehabilitation Centre
180 Woodbridge Street
Fredericton, New Brunswick
Canada E3B-4R3

Julie Shaperman, OT
UCLA Child Amputee Project
Rehabilitation Center
Room 25-26
1000 Veteran Ave.
Los Angeles, CA 90024

Linda Stelzer, OT
Juvenile Amputee Clinic
Detroit Institute for Children
5447 Woodward Avenue
Detroit, MI 48202

INTRODUCTION

Prosthetic treatment options for pediatric upper-limb amputees have expanded in recent years much more rapidly than has useful information on the relative merits of new prosthetic approaches. Clinical decisions have become increasingly complex as a result of lack of research into available treatment methods and prescription components. In addition, no reports of normative prosthetic prehensile function data exist to aid the therapist and other clinic team members in determining appropriate training termination points, assessing treatment efficacy, predicting a child's future prosthetic performance or diagnosing developmental delays.

The absence of pre-school prosthetic performance tests is traceable in part to a paucity of information regarding bimanual activities of daily living skills that may reasonably be expected of **non-amputee** children but which can be performed with a prosthesis. Such information would provide at least tentative guidelines for creating assessment tools for rehabilitation of child amputees at various developmental levels and ages. The presence of prosthetic tests for adults (e.g., Kay and Peizer, 1958) may also have inhibited creative test development efforts devoted to child amputees; however, tests for adults are not easily adapted to assessment of the pre-school amputee. The paucity of pediatric prosthetic prehension assessments must stem in part from the general difficulty found in testing children with any standardized performance instrument. Happily, these general difficulties are no more a barrier to testing amputee children than to testing non-amputee children. Whatever the reason, no such test exists. This symposium was convened in part to redress that shortcoming.

The purpose of the Pre-School Prehension Evaluation Symposium was to bring together expert therapists experienced in pediatric upper-limb amputee rehabilitation, to begin the process of developing a test battery for assessment of prosthetic prehension performance among very young children. The purpose of this book is to record the conceptual background of the Symposium, present the day's deliberations, and expose our thinking to the cold light of day so that others may profit from, criticize, and expand upon the efforts invested in this endeavor.

Each year the Association of Children's Prosthetic-Orthotic Clinics (ACPOC) brings together at its annual convention clinicians concerned with the treatment of orthopedically disabled children. (For more information, contact the ACPOC Secretariat, NYU Prosthetics and Orthotics, 317 East 34th Street, New York, NY 10016, (212) 340-6677.) For the past several years myoelectric and body-powered hands for unilateral upper-limb deficient children have generated the greatest interest during the clinical presentation portions of that meeting. Unfortunately, little hard scientific data can be brought to bear upon discussion of the merits of hook, hand, or control system options available for treatment of the child amputee. As a result, ACPOC discussions (and the everyday treatment decisions affecting the cases presented) primarily center around anecdotal reports and clinical intuition.

The problem became particularly acute during the ACPOC May 1983 meeting in Salt Lake City, when several new myoelectric and body-powered hand terminal devices were introduced to the participating clinics. At the cocktail party following that day's presentations, a group of therapists agreed that a consensus conference, much like those used by NIH to develop approaches to medical diagnostic problems, was needed. We agreed to discuss the problems of assessing the merits of various terminal devices and training approaches for pre-school amputees.

During the months following that May meeting, it became clear that the scope of such an enterprise must be restricted to permit effective consensus. Because a recent census of ACPOC clinics indicated that unilateral below-elbow deficiencies were by far the most prevalent upper-limb amputations among children (Krebs and Fishman, 1984), the Pre-School Prehension Evaluation Symposium targeted its effort on unilateral below-elbow amputees under age seven. We do not mean to imply that children above age seven may be properly assessed using adult prehension tests; age seven was chosen as our upper age limit as much for convenience of the conferees as for the fact that school attendance brings with it a rapid development in prehension skills. Age two was chosen as the lower limit for consideration, since children under that age are rarely fitted with active upper-limb prostheses. The posts

and passive mits fitted to toddlers cannot actively appre-
hend objects, and so prosthetic prehension skills cannot be
assessed. Chapter I outlines other substantive reasons for
limiting the population under discussion to two to seven
year-olds.

Having defined the objectives of a consensus confer-
ence, a proposal was brought before the ACPOC Executive
Board, who provided partial support for a one-day sympo-
sium to be held April 25, 1984, prior to that year's Annual
Meeting in Baltimore. Dr. Scott Decker, Clinic Chief at
James L. Kernan Hospital, agreed to host the Prehension
Symposium. We are grateful to the ACPOC Executive
Board and Dr. Decker for providing a meeting room and
other services at no cost during the Symposium.

Nineteen ACPOC therapists who had substantial experience in the treatment (and in several cases, research)
of pre-school unilateral below-elbow amputees were invited to participate in the Symposium. The fifteen participants are listed on pp. vii-ix. Each was asked to submit
bimanual, repetitive tasks that could be developed into
test items, and ultimately be included in a battery of age-
appropriate functional assessments. In addition, each was
asked to contribute references to help develop a comprehensive bibliography. The compiled bimanual tasks are
listed in Appendix A.

Following four oral presentations (Chapters I, 2, 3,
and 4), the task list was presented to the participants.
Each item was discussed and evaluated by the group as a
whole to ensure that the task could be performed repeti-
tively and bimanually by amputees. The group then esti-
mated the lowest age at which a child with "average"
prosthetic competence could be expected to perform each
item on the list.

Roughly five tasks were chosen for each two year age
span (ages two to three, four to five, and six to seven) to
be included in the final test battery. Operational defini-
tions, starting and finishing positions, and scoring criteria
for each of the tasks were specified by subgroups of the
Symposium participants. The assessment batteries and
scoring criteria were then presented to the other Symposium participants for criticism and refinement.

Upon conclusion of the symposium, each participant
agreed to critically apply the assessment batteries to
children in his/her local clinic. Comments and criticisms

based on these empirical experiences with approximately 50 children have been incorporated into the test batteries presented in Appendix C. While this procedure is hardly systematic or scientific, it was the only available method for gaining insight into the empirical validity of the test items, given our limited monetary resources. Having been subjected to consensual validity analysis at the Symposium and limited empirical testing in the weeks following, it is unlikely that the tests contain egregious errors, but they can not yet be considered scientifically valid or reliable. That undertaking is left to the future.

David E. Krebs, PhD, PT
Editor

Chapter 1

Susan Dustin Clarke, MA, OTR

PREHENSION AND DEVELOPMENTAL THEORY: REVIEW OF NORMAL SKILLS ACQUISITION

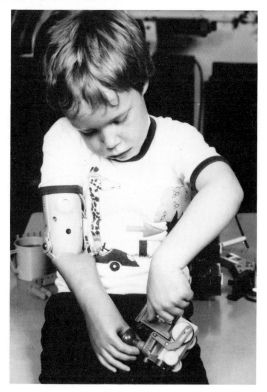

Acquisition of normal prehensile skills is dependent upon many factors. Development of these prehensile skills arises from a summation of many other aspects of child development. The purpose of this chapter is to describe the development of prehensile skills and their interrelationships with four other developmental skills: gross motor development, hand function, hand dominance, and adaptive/cognitive development. This discussion is limited to the child between the ages of eight months and five years. Also considered is the relationship between the development of prehensile skills (and the mastery of other developmental skills) and the ability of a child with a limb deficiency to use and integrate a below-elbow prosthesis into his or her daily activities.

Gross motor development refers to the human process of conquering gravity, including the development of posture and movement strategies that permit purposeful action. In the normal individual gross motor development is primarily a process of maturation, dependent on the status of postural reflexes (Gilfoyle, Grady, and Moore, 1981).

Development of hand function is also primarily maturational, although lack of opportunity to practice can delay development. The evolution of hand function can be tracked by identifying the types of grasp patterns present at different stages of development. These grasp patterns are well documented in the literature on the development of hand function (Erhardt, 1982).

Adaptive/cognitive development encompasses certain aspects of development that are related to purposeful activity when it is defined as the ability to organize behaviors in a manner that allows adaptation and incorporation of new experiences into useful actions. Adaptive/cognitive development includes the integration of perceptions and thoughts into patterns of action, and reflects both maturational and environmental experiences (Maier, 1965).

Development of hand dominance is an aspect of the developmental process that has an interesting and significant effect on prehensile skills acquisition. Humans show a preference for performing most unilateral and fine prehensile tasks with either the left or the right hand. This preference develops over the first eight years of life. Gesell et al. (1940), in studies of development, identified

3

variations in patterns of hand dominance at specific stages of development. The effects of these variations can be seen in the development of both prehensile skills and hand function. They also appear to have a significant influence on the early development of the child's functional use of his or her prosthesis, both as a unit and as a prehensile device.

The interrelationships among these four developmental skills and the development of prehensile function are best illustrated by discussing specific developmental stages of life and identifying the effects of each skill at each stage. Eight stages of life from eight months to five years of age have been selected to illustrate the changing relationships between developmental tasks and the acquisition of prehensile skills.

THE EIGHT MONTH-OLD

The major gross motor task of eight month-old infants is to begin to overcome gravity (Gilfoyle, Grady, and Moore, 1981). By eight months babies learn to maintain an upright sitting posture, thus freeing their hands to explore the environment around them. They are able to grasp and manipulate objects with both hands, or to reach and grasp with one hand while the other assists in balance and body support. The eight month-old begins to use a gross palmar grasp; the thumb is combined with the first two fingers to grasp objects securely. Controlled release also begins at this time. This is significant since it allows the child to serially investigate objects even while one hand is occupied in providing balance and support (Erhardt, 1982).

These infants demonstrate many gains in cognitive/ adaptive behavior. They are able to assimilate new experiences and use what they have learned to augment and expand existing behavior patterns. This assimilation is reinforced by infants' improving ability to track objects visually (Pulaski, 1978).

At this stage hand dominance is expressed as a preference for mixed, unilateral hand use. Because one hand is called upon to provide body support or balance and the other hand is free to explore objects, hand preference for a given activity is dependent on the direction of the pull of gravity which compels upper-limb support on one side or

4

the other (Erhardt, 1982).

The eight month-old with a below-elbow limb deficiency can use a prosthesis effectively to aid in providing body support, as well as to clasp large objects or stabilize smaller ones, while the sound hand is used to explore them. Use of the prosthesis to provide balance and body support allows and encourages the unilateral development of prehension through serial exploration of objects (Clarke and Patton, 1980).

THE FIFTEEN MONTH-OLD

At fifteen months most toddlers have mastered gravity; they are upright and mobile. The mastery of gross motor skills no longer impinges on free use of the hands to explore and manipulate the environment. Ability to manipulate objects is improved markedly. Most fifteen month-olds are capable of refined pincer grasp between finger tips or finger nails, with the distal joint of the thumb flexed. Release is well-controlled, allowing the child to place a pellet in a small container. They have become proficient simple tool users, and can use crayons to scribble and spoons to feed themselves quite neatly (Erhardt, 1982).

The cognitive/adaptive skills of fifteen month-olds are closely linked to eye-hand coordination. They seem impelled to manually explore everything they see. At the same time, fifteen month-olds are developing the ability to grasp objects outside the visual field. Attention span is greatly improved, and the fascination with manipulating small toys and objects makes it easy to engage these children in simple, yet specific tasks. Interest in fine motor activities encourages unilateral dominance. The dominant hand is most often used to manipulate an object, while the non-dominant hand is passive or acts as a holder or stabilizer (Erhardt, 1982; Fraiberg, 1959; Pulaski, 1978).

The fifteen month-old amputee wearing a below-elbow prosthesis will tolerate having objects placed in the terminal device by parent or therapist. Curiosity about objects in general, and a strong desire to manipulate them, usually distracts the amputee from the otherwise vociferous objections to having the prosthesis handled. At fifteen months use of newly acquired prehensile skills

5

through manual manipulation of objects has a high priority, and there are few activities that will engage these children with greater enthusiasm (Clarke and Patton, 1980).

THE EIGHTEEN MONTH-OLD

At eighteen months of age children seem caught between stages of development. Although hand function and coordination have improved enough for them to be capable of manipulating most objects and tools, they lack the cognitive/adaptive skills necessary to use the objects to their fullest potential. Prehensile skills, especially grasp and release, continue to be refined. Use of a fisted tool grasp, and use of the entire upper-limb as a unit, are also more advanced than in fifteen month-olds. Practice allows the eighteen month-old to draw a line and to stack blocks accurately. Just emerging are the cognitive/adaptive abilities that will allow the eighteen month-old to look for cause-and-effect, follow two-step directions, and fit two parts of a puzzle together. Also developing is a greater interest in the effects of their own actions on the environment around them (Erhardt, 1982; Maier, 1965).

The combination of increased motor skills and curiosity about the effects of their actions on the environment causes the eighteen month-old to flit from one activity to another. Newly developed skills are used to approach tasks in new and changing ways. The ability to concentrate is inconsistent because interests are too diversified; these children are unable to predict the outcomes of their actions, since the sense of cause-and-effect is not well developed. The eighteen month-old's internal focus is on the act; the result is often a surprise (Erhardt, 1982; Fraiberg, 1959; Maier, 1965).

Prior to age two upper-limb dominance patterns are a jumble of bilateral and unilateral hand use, with variability in the hand chosen to perform traditionally dominant tasks. These children experiment with varying hand use patterns as part of exercising their curiosity with cause-and-effect. Increased coordination and skill levels make such experimentation possible (Erhardt, 1982).

An eighteen month-old with below-elbow limb deficiency will continue to use a prosthesis as an assisting limb. Although new prehensile skills have developed in the

6

sound hand, these changes are primarily the result of neuromuscular maturation. Prehensile function is best facilitated by the amputee experimenting with growing awareness of cause-and-effect. Formal training programs are usually not successful at this time, due to the eighteen month-old's need to exercise independence in exploration of the environment. They are not motivated by the consistency of results of a training program, because they are unable to predict outcome; their interest is captivated by the often surprising results of their own experimentation on the environment around them (Fraiberg, 1957; Gilfoyle, Grady, and Moore, 1981; Maier, 1965).

THE TWO YEAR-OLD

The major developmental milestone for two year-olds is the mastery of simple reasoning. In addition, more complex gross motor skills such as tricycle riding are developing. Fine motor skills and function continue to improve, as illustrated by changing grasp patterns. A more refined grip, in which a tool is held with the fingers rather than in the fist, develops. The wrist is held in neutral flexion/extension, and in slight ulnar deviation. The forearm still moves as a unit, which allows more control and coordination during tool use (Erhardt, 1982).

Prehensile and cognitive skill advances allow the two year-old to accomplish such diverse tasks as jumping in place, throwing a ball overhand, and assembling put-together toys. They also allow the child to use these skills in simple organized play that combines more than one task. Dominance patterns shift to unilateral use of the dominant hand, giving two year-olds the maximum benefit of their newly acquired fine dexterity (Erhardt, 1982).

At this stage, primitive reasoning and delayed memory also make possible the development of speech. Thus, two year-olds can plan ahead and focus on the outcome that a particular action will produce. The improved understanding of cause-and-effect allows them to predict the results of their actions (Maier, 1965). Because reasoning is simplistic, two year-olds often use faulty logic to reach conclusions about the expected outcomes of their actions. This faulty logic, combined with a growing sense of self, helps to create the period of development often

7

referred to as the "terrible twos" (Fraiberg, 1959). Because the two year-old is finally able to organize simple tasks into a many-step task with a forseeable outcome, this age is an ideal time to introduce a formal training program for children with below-elbow limb deficiencies.

Two year-old amputees are readily able to master operation of active terminal devices, and to apply these skills to simple functional activities. Newly acquired memory skills permit prosthetic skills to be generalized to diverse activities, thus increasing the opportunity for practical use of the prosthesis in everyday activities. They have the ability to focus on a new task, take instruction, and complete the task. The attention span of the two year-old, augmented by a growing understanding of cause-and-effect and the ability to reason and remember, allows them to anticipate end results, and thus allows prosthetic training to be effective (Clarke, 1982; Clarke and Patton, 1980; Pulaski, 1978).

THE THREE YEAR-OLD

At three years of age fine motor skills improve rapidly. Expanded abilities to problem-solve and to understand what makes things work, coupled with increased neuromotor maturity, allow three year-olds to interact with the environment on a more sophisticated level. Their curiosity is piqued by a new understanding of how the world works. Language usage now reflects a new grasp of adverbs and analogies, as well as the ability to define words. Changes in cognitive processes are also reflected in the way three year-olds use their hands. They are very bilateral in their approach to tasks. They may alternate the hand used as dominant, and they approach the same task in many different ways. It is as if they need to try all possibilities so they can select the approach which is most effective (Erhardt, 1982; Maier, 1965; Pulaski, 1978).

Prehensile skills, although improved over those of the two year-old, are still immature, as demonstrated by pencil grasp. The three year-old uses a static tripod hold with the wrist in a neutral position, allowing only gross control of the pencil (Erhardt, 1982).

For below-elbow amputees, age three to four is a period of increased reliance on the prosthesis for assistance in bimanual activities. The terminal device of the prosthesis is used frequently as a grasping tool because of the high demand for bimanual exploration of small objects and the relatively low dexterity of the sound hand. Task performance and completion, however, is inconsistent, due to the level of experimentation and exploration that commonly goes on at this age. Although a new task may be completed successfully, it may not be completed in the same fashion on a second trial (Clarke and Patton, 1980; Erhardt, 1982).

THE FOUR YEAR-OLD

By age four children develop a social interest in the world around them. They begin to understand relationships between objects in the immediate environment, but may still misperceive those that are distant or abstract. For example, although four year-olds may understand that a toy sailboat moves because of wind blowing the sails, they may still believe that clouds are alive because they move (Fraiberg, 1959).

They also have gained skills in self-care. They like this new feeling of independence and prefer to do things for themselves. Because of their growing social awareness, four year-olds desire approval from adults. They will follow instructions, but do best when allowed some independence in deciding how to accomplish a task (Fraiberg, 1959; Pulaski, 1978).

At age four children progress toward development of a mature unilateral dominance pattern, due to improved coordination in the preferred hand. Amputees of this age are more likely to be consistent in use of the prosthesis as an assisting limb compared to themselves at three years of age (Erhardt, 1982).

THE FIVE YEAR-OLD

By five years of age children reach a plateau in gross motor development. Motor skills are now excellent and spontaneous. Energy previously invested in developing basic motor skills can now be used to improve and expand existing skills (Gilfoyle, Grady, and Moore, 1981).

Hand function improves through practice. By the end of the fifth year all basic prehensile skills are present, as illustrated by the acquisition of an adult pencil grip using a dynamic tripod posture with precise opposition of the thumb, index finger, and middle finger. The wrist is held slightly extended, and the pencil is grasped near the lead. Consistent unilateral hand preference is usually well-established in the five year-old, and the non-dominant extremity assumes a more passive role in assisting with bimanual activities (Erhardt, 1982).

At this stage of development, adaptive/cognitive behavior becomes more advanced. Although far from mature, the thought processes of five year-olds have moved from the preconceptual phase of development into the phase of intuitive-preoperational thought. Thus, the scaffolding is erected upon which operational thought will build at about the seventh year of life (Maier, 1965).

From age five development of prehensile skills becomes a direct function of experience and practice. As maturation peaks, growth and practice account for further development of grasp size and dexterity. Dominance is well established, and its effects on prehension patterns remain consistent (Erhardt, 1982).

Lack of operational thought in the five year-old amputee impedes prosthetic training and use. These children are unable to fully understand the relationships between objects and actions. Although the child may verbally employ relational expressions, he or she may not fully understand the conceptual relationship thus expressed. The five year-old amputee typically questions those around him about growth of the residual limb, especially if finger buds or nubbins are present. The child may erroneously compare the growth of seeds into plants with the potential growth of his nubbins into fingers or a hand (Maier, 1965; Pulaski, 1978).

Similar faulty logic may lead to misinterpretation of cause-and-effect. Children may blame the prosthesis for failure to complete a task accurately, as if the device were animate. If parents and therapists are aware of these age-related normal flaws in logic, they can assist the child by not interpreting his reactions as signs of emotional problems, but instead helping to develop a more realistic understanding of the situation at the child's level of reasoning.

SUMMARY

Interrelationships among normal prehensile skills acquisition and gross motor development, development of hand function, adaptive/cognitive development, and hand dominance have been presented at various stages of development. The effects of such relationships on the development of prosthetic skills by unilateral below-elbow amputees have also been discussed. Steps in growth and development, maturation, and prehensile skills acquisition are closely linked to each other and to the potential success of prosthetic fitting and training for the child with a below-elbow limb deficiency.

The relationships among these developmental tasks should guide the construction of prosthetic prehension tests, the evaluation of treatment programs, and the design of prosthetic components for the young amputee. The effect of developmental status on each subject tested must be considered in every aspect of the procedure. Selection of test items, test environment, instruction format, and test item duration are just a few of the procedures affected by developmental status. The task of developing tests and evaluations, particularly for two to five year-old children in various developmental stages, is a most complex problem because of the continually changing diversity of abilities present throughout early childhood.

11

Chapter 2

David E. Krebs, PhD, PT

TEST AND MEASUREMENT THEORY RELEVANT TO ULP PERFORMANCE

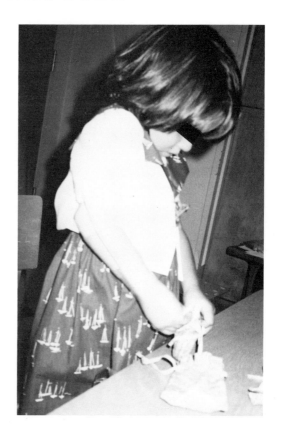

Pediatric unilateral below-elbow amputee prosthetic performance assessment must comply with the principles governing any scientific inquiry. Tests complying with these criteria may then be useful for investigation into treatment approaches, comparison of prosthetic components, development of normative prosthetic prehension performance data, diagnosis of developmental delays, prediction of future prosthetic performance, determination of training efficacy or completion criteria, and evaluation of other factors affecting amputee functional rehabilitation. Each test purpose determines the details of design and application, but several factors are common to any prosthetic performance test. This chapter describes the principal elements of a useful test, specifically relating these elements to quantitative prosthetic prehension test batteries.

Good clinical tests are comprehensive, feasible in a clinical setting, and sensitive to changes in the subject's performance. To be comprehensive, a prosthetic prehension assessment battery should contain a variety of items (tasks) that represent the range of prosthetic use in everyday life. Task performance is measured in a clinic; it is these measures -- not real-life events -- that are analyzed. To generate useful information, a prosthetic performance test must reflect as closely as possible a given subject's prosthetic prehension behavior in life. In short, a pediatric prehension test battery must reflect real Activities of Daily Living (ADL) requirements of the test population at a given age. The three most important elements of test design are measurement technique, reliability of the items, and validity of the battery as a whole.

MEASUREMENT

Measurement is the assignment of numbers to events according to rules. The rules link the investigator's concepts (the assumptions of the test battery) to concrete arithmetic notations which can be analyzed and interpreted. Measurement in prosthetic prehension tests may link abstract ideas to numbers. For example, developmental age or perceptual, cognitive, and motor skills may be linked to numeric indices of the quality or speed of prosthetic use. Specifically, one tester might rate the ability of amputees to cut a complex shape from a piece of paper, and use this to assess cognitive development. Measurement may also link concrete factors to numeric indices; a tester might use the same shape-cutting task to assess ADL skills.

To enable measurements to reflect the conceptual interests of the designers of the test, the operational rules used by the raters must be precisely defined. One cannot naively assign numbers to behaviors and expect the measurements to be meaningful. The most difficult (but potentially the most interesting) aspect of measurement is the rule by which the numbers are assigned. Examples of rules governing prosthetic assessment include the following:

"When does the test begin and end?"
"What are the rater and subject positions during the test?"
"What instructions are given to the subject?"
"What constitutes successful completion of the test?
"When should a trial be judged invalid and therefore ignored?"
"When should the trial be repeated?"

In short, measurement is the most basic of test requirements. The test's operational rules should be consistent with the tester's assumptions, because to a great extent it is these rules that determine the meaning of test scores.

RELIABILITY

Reliability is simply accuracy -- the extent to which a test yields similar results on repeated trials. Reliable tests are absolutely fundamental to obtaining meaningful, interpretable clinical data. Ideally variations in test scores should be due only to differences in the underlying factor being examined (e.g., a prosthetic treatment); unfortunately, error is also an ever-present source of test score differences.

Statistical determinations of reliability are based upon the following principle: Some (usually unknown) proportion of the final score is due to error, and some portion is due to real differences. Exhaustive exploration of this important principle is, however, beyond the scope of this chapter. Those interested are referred to any good statistical text for further information on the mathematics of reliability analysis (for example, Edward G. Carmines and Richard A. Zeller: Reliability and Validity Assessment. Beverly Hills, CA: Sage, 1979). The important message is that designers of test batteries must acknowledge and attempt to minimize the effects of test error. Test error limits test reliability.

The reliability of a clinical test depends primarily upon measurement accuracy and performance consistency.

Measurement Reliability

Reliable (accurate) tests are characterized by unambiguous testing instructions and a consistent testing environment; these permit the test to be administered identically with different children, or with the same child at different times, independent of the tester's mood or other status at the time of testing.

Prehension test measurement reliability rests upon three principles:

1. Define the task's operational rules clearly and administer each item consistently.
2. Provide clear and standard instructions to each subject.
3. Increase the number of test items if reliability is in doubt.

Each tester must operate under the same rules as the other testers; for example, each task must have unambiguous beginning and end points, and each tester must score the observed behaviors consistently. Each tester must provide the same instructions by saying the same words and giving the same amount of help to each subject. To understand the third principle (increasing the number of test items when reliability is in doubt), recall the last time you measured a distance with a ruler; if you were not sure the resulting length was accurate, you repeated the measurement, perhaps with a different ruler, to increase your accuracy.

17

Performance Reliability

In addition to measurement reliability, meaningful testing requires performance reliability. That is, not only must the testers score the observed behaviors consistently, but the test subjects must also be able to perform the tests similarly if they are retested. In many scientific investigations (e.g., determination of the maze-solving abilities of rats) performance reliability is assumed, provided that the test is administered with the same rules under all conditions (i.e., the subjects are given the same instructions, motivation, and amount of help during each test). Clinical trials, particularly those seeking to test children, must grapple with the complex problem of subject inconsistency. Whereas enhancing measurement reliability focuses upon decreasing the foibles of the rater, improving performance reliability seeks to decrease the idiosyncratic contributions of the subject's mood and other ephemeral factors unimportant to the resulting test scores.

Prosthetic tests have in the past been scored either by timing a test item, or by judging the quality of prehension performance, but little attention has been paid to the reliability of each method. Although there are no published empirical data to support the following claims, logic and my clinical experience indicate that both scoring schemes have assets and liabilities.

It seems reasonable to assert that timing the performance of a child opening a series of nested kegs has high measurement reliability but moderate performance reliability, depending as it does upon the prior experience, motivation, attention, and interest of the child both in completing the task and doing so as rapidly as possible. Ratings of the quality of the child's prosthetic skills in extracting these same kegs may suffer less from performance inconsistency, because the child is not necessarily constrained to perform the task in a standardized, rapid, and perhaps unnatural fashion; the child need only be interested in completing the task. Furthermore, raters can suspend judgment when the child is obviously not attending to the task. However, measurement reliability suffers when using a qualitative scale, because no one has been able to define prosthetic performance quality in a way that

18

is simultaneously meaningful, precise, and accurate over a variety of test situations.

Designing test procedures so that the items can be performed as naturally as possible will reduce the tendency of children not to attend to an obviously artificial and perhaps boring task. If task performance can be totally standardized without introducing excessive artificiality, then quantifying the results by timing the duration of the test event is probably preferable. If, however, the tester is interested in the quality of prosthetic performance (such as determining spontaneous prehension problem-solving skills), then descriptive scales must be developed and extensively tested for measurement reliability and stability over raters. In the latter case, quantitative analysis is not the goal, so no further attention will be given to such tests in this chapter.

To summarize, prehension test scores cannot be useful unless they represent a realistic, stable measure of the amputee's prosthetic skills. The extent to which the resultant data represent temporary conditions peculiar to that tester, test situation, or the amputee's fleeting mood, is the extent to which the test results err in providing a stable determination of prosthetic performance. The degree to which the tester requires quantitative data determines the scale construction; timed tests are exemplary for their potential measurement reliability, but test validity may be compromised if too many concessions to artificiality must be made during the necessary task standardization.

VALIDITY

The extent to which an item measures what it purports to measure is its validity. In pediatric prosthetic prehension assessment it is important that most children be able to complete the tasks, and that the tasks are those which a child of average competence at a given age would usually perform with a prosthesis. That is, the task must be as close as possible to things that would be done in real life. For example, we may believe that we are measuring the prehension agility of an amputee when we determine how long the child takes to open a package of crackers, but if the subject has no experience with cellophane we may in

19

fact be measuring intelligence or ability to solve spatial orientation tasks. Indeed, if the amputee is two years old, this task may not be measuring anything but trial-and-error. This important concept is called isomorphism (literally "similarity of form") between the test and reality. The extent to which a task reflects reality is its degree of veridicality or isomorphism. The remainder of this chapter describes three tenets of prehension test item validity for unilateral pediatric below-elbow amputees: Tasks should be bimanual, repetitive, and age-appropriate.

Bimanuality

No unilateral amputee will use the terminal device (TD) for unilateral tasks. Given that prosthetic functional tests, in general, should reflect activities an amputee would be likely to perform in real life, it follows that the test items should compel bimanual prehension. For example, a unilateral upper-limb amputee would not normally use the TD to pick up jelly-beans from a table-top; in real life the sound hand would be employed. Therefore, test batteries that assess prosthetic jelly-bean transfers from a table-top to a container are not isomorphic with reality.

Repetition

Opening and closing the TD in a variety of positions will most closely reflect general prosthetic prehension skill (Gilad, 1985). To measure prehension skill, a test should concentrate on repetitive grasping. In normal use, of course, the TD may be employed for a variety of non-prehensile activities, such as pushing and pulling items or acting as a static paperweight. Non-repetitive or non-prehensile tests, however, probably reflect non-prosthetic factors such as gross motor agility.

A test item's ability to discriminate between levels of performance derives in part from the task's duration (Lehneis, 1975). If the tasks are too brief or excessively long, variability in test scores will result from chance or factors that are otherwise unrelated to real prehension skills. A task that takes only three seconds to perform or is excessively simple would also generate variability due only to chance. For example, testing an amputee's ability to simply grasp one item from a table and place it in a box could not discriminate levels of prosthetic prehension skill; errors such as not focusing immediately on the task would contribute disproportionately during scoring, and would outweigh the legitimate information that could be contained in the scores. Similar logic holds for a task which takes too long to perform; the subjects, especially young children, will become bored and stop attending during a very long trial. Therefore, each task should be repetitive and of sufficient duration to generate legitimate variability in the test scores to discriminate factors of interest.

Age-Appropriateness

Each test item must reflect skills an amputee would be expected to possess at a given age. As indicated above, chance variability will dominate the test scores if the items are too easy or too difficult. The choice of proper test items to discriminate between levels of prehension performance is clear-cut only at the extremes; it would be just as obviously invalid to test an eighteen year-old on a battery of paper-tearing and crayon-coloring items as to test a three year-old on a battery of wood-working items.

Unfortunately, few bimanual prehension tasks have been age-standardized for normal children. Appendix A presents a task list generated by participants of the Symposium; each task was age-estimated by the participants. One method of developing age-appropriate test items is to draw upon the clinical experience of experts, such as those attending the Symposium, to synthesize their experiences with whatever data exist on normal subjects (Chapter I includes an overview of normal prehension). Clearly, amputees cannot be expected to exceed performance standards of their two-handed peers; therefore, a primary task is to determine the prehension decrement caused by amputation and prosthetic restoration. Projections of task age-appropriateness for below-elbow amputees must synthesize knowledge of amputee developmental skill levels and a realistic assessment of prevailing prostheses and training techniques.

Assessment of age-appropriateness is also difficult for mathematical reasons. Age is a continuum, but the practicalities of test administration force us to construct non-continuous (discrete) test batteries: one test for two to three year-old children, another for four to five year-olds, and so on. In addition, chronological age may not be the best criterion for dividing the subjects into test groups.

21

Some very mature three year-olds will find the youngsters' test too easy, and some four year-olds will find the four to five year-olds' test too hard. One approach is to make many tests, one for each six month age span; by so doing, we might gain test specificity. A better approach might be to use a pretest to divide the children into skill levels, and then perform the prosthetic prehension test.

For example, standardized motor milestones could be employed as the pretest. Perhaps a gross motor test, such as duration of one-legged balance, might be helpful: two seconds is standard for unilateral stance in four year-olds, three seconds for five year-olds, and more than ten seconds for seven year-olds. A fine motor test of the sound hand may be even more related to prehension performance; the ability to stack three blocks could be defined as the standard for a two to three year-olds' test; six to seven stacked blocks would gain admittance to the four to five year-olds' test, and so on (Illingworth, 1975). By administering a pretest one could be more sure that the prosthetic prehension test is appropriate for a given amputee, and thus improve the reliability and validity of that test.

In summary, each test item in a valid prosthetic prehension test for unilateral amputees must compel bilateral, repetitive grasp and release. Approach, TD prepositioning, duration of grasp, spontaneity of use, psychological reactions, and many other factors may also be considered relevant in a comprehensive test battery, but these factors should not be confused with fine prehension skills. Valid prehension tasks are not only age-appropriate and representative of tasks an amputee would be expected to perform in daily living, they are also appropriate for the amputation level and the prosthetic components worn by the subject.

Validity Assessment

There are many ways to determine the validity of test items. One means of determining task validity is to assess the extent to which test items generate clear discriminations between levels of some factor of interest. For example, test battery scores from many children could be compared with some "gold standard" (such as amputee age) to determine the natural groups into which the test items cluster. These clusters might then define the items to be

22

included in amputee prehension tests at a given age.

Perhaps the most convenient method of validity assessment is to set up a list of tasks that amputees commonly perform, and then adapt them to a testing situation. For example, participants in the Symposium judged the prima facie validity of over 50 items (listed in Appendix A). Most of these tasks are bimanual and represent part of the universe of activities that pre-school amputees master during daily living. Symposium participants developed a consensus on items that they believed to be useful for inclusion in a prosthetic prehension assessment battery. This method of validity determination is called "consensual validity."

Of course, adapting the items to test situations introduces a degree of artificiality; simply being closely observed and rated introduces some test anxiety, and the presence of a tester adds an element of unfamiliarity to the amputee's usual environment. Unfortunately, there is no good solution to this problem, so it is typically ignored (in part because each item must be adapted to a standardized test situation to permit reliable measurement). The tester must determine if the standardization has compromised test isomorphism.

The final test should include a variety of activities, each of which should represent a specific domain of prosthetic use. By choosing some items that reflect prosthetic skills during eating, others that tap prehension during dressing, and still others that sample hygiene skills, assessment of the full spectrum of prehension activities for which the prosthesis is used in real life becomes possible, thus enhancing the validity of the test battery as a whole. That is, the validity of each item must be carefully assessed for appropriateness, and the items that make up the test battery should be chosen on the basis of how representative they are of the types of activities such amputees are expected to perform in daily living.

Finally, the subjects must not be permitted to practice the test; prosthetic training must be conducted on tasks that are not included in the test battery. Allowing the participant to practice the test is similar to letting a student obtain a copy of an examination prior to its administration; the test may only reflect how well the participant remembers the pretest experience.

To assert that developing a valid, age-appropriate

prehension assessment battery is a difficult undertaking is to state the obvious. Although the results of the Symposium provide a starting point, we should not presume to have finished our job of test development until the test battery has been empirically evaluated through systematic scrutiny of each item's validity and reliability during assessment of many young amputees.

SUMMARY

No published prosthetic prehension assessment test batteries have been scientifically scrutinized for reliability and validity. The purpose of prehension testing, in a limited sense, is to assign numbers to prosthetic performance. By combining knowledge about normal prehension skill development, amputees' prosthetic utilization, and testing principles, one can choose tasks that are age-appropriate, specify the domain that the items tap, and develop rules for reliably assigning numbers to the test performance.

Prehension tests must be continually refined until they are demonstrated to be valid and optimally comprehensive. The message of this chapter is that our best efforts today must be empirically tested, revised, and refined as more knowledge is obtained about the pre-school amputee population and prosthetic prehension testing methods.

Chapter 3

Sheila Hubbard, PT, OT

PREHENSION AND MOTOR SKILLS TESTING IN CHILD UPPER EXTERMITIES AMPUTEES

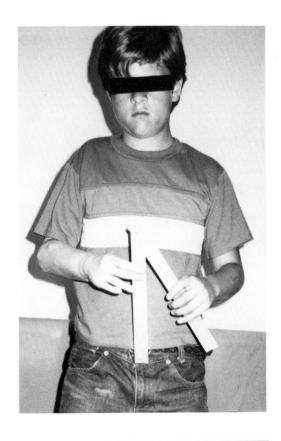

A search of the prosthetic literature of the past twenty years reveals:
1. individual case reports illustrating unusual surgery or fittings;
2. discussion papers with limited data bases;
3. evaluation reports of prosthetic components;
4. a limited number of systematic research reports dealing primarily with adult populations; and
5. very little objective data on upper-limb amputee management or functional achievement.

SYSTEMATIC RESEARCH ON NON-AMPUTEE ADULTS

Over the years there have been a number of attempts to produce standardized tests of normal hand function to permit comparisions among persons with upper extremity impairment. An example of such a test was devised by Jebsen et al. (1969). Seven subtests were chosen to provide a broad sampling of hand function; these activities were timed for both the nondominant and dominant hands. Three hundred subjects were tested, and norms were established for five adult age ranges. The test was then repeated on 26 patients with stable hand disabilities to evaluate test reliability.

A similar project was carried out by Kellor, Frost, and Silberberg (1971). Two hundred and fifty men and women were tested for grip strength and hand dexterity. The norms developed were intended to facilitate comparison of patients with hand disabilities to normal individuals of the same age and sex.

AMPUTEE ASSESSMENT

Adults

Attempts have been made to adapt adult functional tests to amputee performance assessment. For example, an Australian study reported by Agnew and Shannon (1981) used the Minnesota Rate of Manipulation Placing Test (American Guidance Service, 1969) and the Smith Hand Function Unilateral Grasp-Release Procedures (Smith, 1973) to evaluate a myoelectrically controlled prosthesis with a sensory feedback system. Results indicated that the average amputee performance was two to three times slower than the average non-amputee performance. The authors concluded that the validity of the two tests administered was questionable. However, in the absence of a specific test of performance of the myoelectric hand, they felt that some measure was needed to compare amputee function with that of the normal, intact hand.

Another study from Sweden, by Herberts et al. (1980), used the "Quantitative Test of Upper Extremity Function" described by Carroll (1965) as part of the evaluation process in assessing the outcome of their rehabilitation program for 16 amputees fitted with myoelectric prostheses.

Children
With regard to juvenile amputees, most of the literature has focused on the debate over appropriate age of fitting and activation, prosthetic check-out procedures, and the problem of prosthetic acceptance by the child and family. One of the earliest formal studies was a questionnaire by Lambert and Sciora (1959). Upper-limb prosthetic use for 65 juvenile amputees was graded as good, fair, or poor according to the questionnaire response from parents.

Brooks and Shaperman (1965) developed their well-known prosthesis adjustment scale (PAS) as a means of evaluating their program at the Child Amputee Prosthetic Project. Each child was rated in each of the five categories (wearing pattern, operating skill, applied used, maintenance, and acceptance). At the conclusion of their study, it was noted that scores in PAS categories 1, 2, 3, and 5 were closely related to each other. Children receiving a high rating in any given category (with the exception of "maintenance") tended to rate highly in the others as well. It was concluded that the category most closely related to successful fitting at an early age was full-time prosthetic wear.

PERFORMANCE TEST METHODS

In recent years a growing interest in amputee rehabilitation generally and the increasing trend toward

28

costlier electromechanical fittings have led to the need for more specific and objective measures to assess and compare performance in use.

Most attempts to produce such a standardized performance procedure seem to fall into two categories:

1) timed dexterity tests designed to evaluate the patient's technical skills in controlling the prosthesis; and

2) a variety of task lists used in combination with rating scales to evaluate the use of the prosthesis in two-handed activities.

Timed Dexterity Tasks

Stein and Walley (1983) adapted the test procedure of Jebsen et al. to compare amputees who wore either myoelectric or conventional prostheses. The amputees were timed on a series of 8 functional tasks while using either their normal hand, their myoelectric hand, or a cable-controlled hook. Compared to their normal hand, amputees took about two and a half times as long to complete the tasks with a conventional prosthesis, and about five times as long with a myoelectric prosthesis. Despite the slower function, 60% of below-elbow amputees preferred the myoelectric prosthesis.

A second timed dexterity test was used in the United Kingdom trial of the Swedish myoelectric hand for young children (Ingvarsson et al., 1980). It took the form of structured activities covered in the training program. Six tasks were scored on successful achievement within a given time; a puzzle test was administered to determine the time to remove and replace all the pieces. The performance test was not used for comparison between children, but only to determine a competence baseline for each child. Parents found the numerical results to be a useful yardstick by which to gauge their child's progress. The greatest improvement occurred between the "end of training" test and the "first review" test six weeks later.

Rating Scales

A variety of rating scales have been used to judge amputee performance in bilateral Activities of Daily Living (ADL). Rating scales were employed as early as 1961 by Teska and Swinyard of New York University in evaluating the then-new APRL-Sierra No. 1 hand (Teska

29

and Swinyard, 1961). The performance test consisted of five play activities; the child's ability was rated as excellent, satisfactory, or unsatisfactory.

Bergholtz (1976), also of NYU, reported an evaluation of the University of New Brunswick (UNB) myoelectric control system. She tested children (aged eleven to twenty) on a series of 12 activities. A numerical score was assigned to the child's ability to use the conventional and experimental prostheses on each of the activities. She found that prosthetic performance depended on the type of activity tested. The myoelectric unit provided more satisfactory terminal device (TD) function in tasks related to grasping, lifting, and holding large bulky objects; cutting meat; and donning clothes. The quality of TD performance was higher for the conventional prosthesis when fine control was needed, as when grasping a soft, small, or flat object.

Another attempt to evaluate the UNB system was reported by Paciga et al. (1980). Along with questionnaires, a functional evaluation was done. Performance was rated as excellent, good, fair, or poor in a battery of seven bimanual tasks. A similar but longer ADL test for adults was reported by Herberts et al. (1980). Fourteen activities were tested, and the performance of each function was rated as 0-3.

Durance and O'Shea (1981) produced an excellent evaluation protocol while reviewing their management of upper-limb amputees in Kingston, Ontario. A simple bimanual task list was used in conjunction with a five-point scale to rate performance according to amount and spontaneity of prosthetic use. Sanderson (personal communication, 1984) has modified this rating scale for use in her research endeavors at the University of New Brunswick.

Crone (personal communications, 1983-1984) at Alberta Children's Hospital has carried out a single case study comparison of a conventional and a myoelectric fitting on one pre-school age amputee by counting the actual number of passive and active uses of the prosthesis during structured play sessions.

THE OCCC EXPERIENCE

Finally, I would like to share our own experience at the Ontario Crippled Children's Center (OCCC) with a pre-

30

school myoelectric training project. The purpose of the project was to compare the cost-effectiveness of two training protocols. One was a home-based program with the parent as primary trainer, and the other was a center-based program with a therapist as trainer. The evaluation procedure was two-fold. Seven activities were carried out in standardized fashion, and the child's ability and the time taken to accomplish the tasks were recorded. The complete session was simultaneously recorded on videotape, and an outside evaluator rated the videotaped activities on a scale of 0-5. The complete test was carried out four times -- initially with the child's conventional prosthesis and then at each of the three review periods following the fitting of the myoelectric device.

Originally we had anticipated using the timed-accomplishment data to demonstrate progress. However, it soon became apparent that this information was not very reliable for young children. The factors of motivation, concentration, concept of time, and problems with battery and prosthetic malfunction varied with each child and with each testing situation. However, the data from the video tests was analyzed statistically. The total test scores for the two groups were compared at each of the four trials; also, the groups' conventional prosthesis scores were compared with the scores at the time of the six month myoelectric follow-up review.

The testing procedure itself was found to be useful, but still requires modification. There were a number of unforeseen variables (such as each child's ability to adjust to the weight of the prosthesis and variations in individual problem-solving ability) which made it difficult to standardize the ratings. Prosthetic complications also occurred during the testing sessions, including batteries running down and new gloves not being stretched enough to allow for maximum opening of the hand. The task list itself was not ideal. Some items did not yield enough information, while others were more repetitious than necessary. The procedure was also too lengthy for the younger subjects. The rating scale itself was too complex and not always appropriate.

More importantly, the test only evaluated directed technical use of the prosthesis, and did not cover the desired spontaneous use of the prosthesis during bimanual activities. It may be of interest to note that in follow-up

31

clinic reviews we have observed that several of the children failed to incorporate the prosthesis into bilateral play activities, despite their ability to demonstrate excellent technical control skill when asked.

SUMMARY

To summarize, it is quite obvious that so far no one has managed to produce an ideal prosthetic evaluation tool for children. While numerous attempts have been made to assess prosthetic skill (by either timed repetitive tasks or ratings of bimanual ADL tasks) no test standardization has occurred. The absence of a valid functional test hampers research efforts universally.

Let me conclude with some words of advice from Teska and Swinyard (1961):

"Tasks designed for children should be as simple and short as possible. Effort must be made to make the test as interesting and as much fun as possible. Tests should be in accord with the child's chronological age and should be applicable to both boys and girls. All the processes involved should be familiar to the child. The clinic environment and the understanding of the child (are) as important as the test itself. Finally, the child should never be pressured to perform successfully."

Chapter 4

Felice Celikyol, MA, OTR

COMPARISON OF TERMINAL DEVICES AND BODY-POWERED/MYOELECTRIC PROSTHETIC SYSTEMS AVAILABLE FOR PRE-SCHOOL UPPER-LIMB AMPUTEES

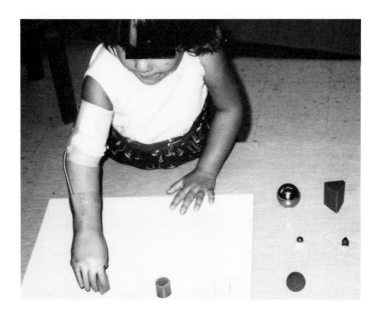

This chapter provides a review of the relevant literature, as well as examining the design features of currently available terminal devices. Myoelectric and body powered systems for two to seven year-old below-elbow (BE) amputees are reviewed in Table 4-1. Table 4-2 provides a feature-by-feature functional comparison of available devices and systems. This information has been gleaned from my clinical experience.

LITERATURE REVIEW

No systematic comparisons of terminal devices and prosthetic systems were found in the literature. The only article that compares body-powered (BP) with myoelectric (M) prostheses on a population close to the two to five year-old age range was published by Trost in 1983.

Trost (1983) examined comfort, appearance, and function, including speed of operation, ease of control, utilization, and energy expended in 45 children, ages six to sixteen. Of the 45 below-elbow amputees studied, 35 wore BP hook prostheses prior to receiving M prostheses with Otto Bock hands. The children were evenly divided in their judgments of which prothesis they considered faster, which they prefered for utilization in daily activities, and which required more energy to operate. Trost notes that there was an overall preference for the myoelectric limb's appearance and comfort, but no difference related to function; overall, the M prosthesis was worn more often than was the BP device.

Gloves and batteries were the two items most often needing repair or replacement, followed by the hand frame and thumb axis. The electrical system needed repairs infrequently, but required longer "down" time. Trost prefers to fit children with myoelectric protheses at age ten and over, stating that younger children are less concerned with cosmesis and therefore less cautious regarding breakage.

Stein and Walley (1983) compared sixteen amputees using BP hooks with twenty users of M hands. The thirty-six subjects were primarily adults, but at least two children under age sixteen were included in the study. Of the sixteen users of BP hooks, ten were below-elbow amputees, and none had myoelectric experience. Fourteen of the twenty M hand users were below-elbow amputees, and all had experience with BP systems. Range of motion, speed, lift, function, and endurance were assessed with

1) standardized performance tests (Jebsen et al., 1969), and
2) Activities of Daily Living questionnaires.

Timed performance tests with M protheses averaged twice as long as with BP systems, and five times as long as with normal limbs. Although tasks were accomplished faster with hooks than with hands, extreme body movements (such as trunk rotation to turn a heavy object) were required during use of the BP hooks because of harnessing constraints. Also, those subjects using BP limbs were unable to open their hooks behind the neck and back as often as M users could. With regard to function, M prostheses were found to be heavier but preferred to BP prostheses, in part due to the freedom from the BP's harness. Appearance of the M hand was preferred to that of the BP hook. Sixty percent of the myoelectric users preferred the M to the BP prothesis.

Feedback

Northmore-Ball, Heger, and Hunter (1980) compared users of the Otto Bock M hand to users of BP hand and hook prostheses. Although the subjects studied were injured workmen and therefore little related to the two to five year-old population, the workmen's comments regarding sensory feedback are of interest. Twenty-three percent of those using BP limbs experienced feedback through cable tension and position of the BP harness (the traditionally accepted concept), while thirty-three percent of those using M limbs emphatically declared that the myoelectric prothesis gave more feedback. The authors attribute the myoelectric users' surprising comments to the more intimate socket of the M prothesis, and to the more "natural" use of muscle control.

Sorbye (1977, 1980) also mentions sensory feedback from myoelectric prostheses. Some two to five year-old children were able to grasp delicate items without using visual feedback. Teenagers, however, tested using UBN 1-site control systems with Otto Bock M hands at the Ontario Crippled Children's Center did not feel confident with feedback from the myoelectric hand for pinch force control (Paciga et al., 1980).

Training

O'Shea and Dunfield (1983) studied 16 normal (no limb deformities) pre-school children aged three to four and a half years. They set out to support the hypothesis that myoelectrically controlled toys would prove to be a more appropriate means for training pre-school children in myoelectric control than would the myotrainer, which offers feedback of an abstract nature. They also compared the ease with which normal children learn to control 1-site and 2-site myoelectric systems. Results supported the use of toys as being more effective because the children showed more interest and were more attentive to toys than to the myotrainer.

The authors suggest that data analysis should focus on accuracy and number of trials at each session as a better measure of training efficiency, rather than on time ratio, which is the time attended to the task divided by the total session time (free play plus training). They caution us on accepting time ratio results since the length of actual training time and play time are difficult to control in this type of testing situation. They further suggest that re-search be directed toward refining training strategies. No significant difference in accuracy rate was found with either the 1-site or 2-site systems.

Lamb and Scott (1981) state that they were much encouraged by their experience in training pre-school amputee children to use M prostheses; they specifically comment on the ease with which items can be grasped and released in a variety of positions relative to the body, as compared with the BP limb.

Sorbye (1977, 1980) states that acceptance of the M prosthesis seems to be better in children than in adults, and advocates fitting amputees prior to age two. Among the advantages of M protheses cited, Sorbye mentions the ability to grasp objects in all upper-limb positions, and the fact that use of muscle contraction prevents atrophy and thus enhances socket retention. He admits that fitting procedures can be very time-consuming, and notes that mechanical maintenance reliability is questionable for the child-sized hand.

37

CASE REPORTS

Our experience in training pre-school children in the use of M prostheses at the Kessler institute is limited. Two recently-fitted, representative children are described below.

The first case, a five year-old boy, was originally fitted with a BP supracondylar below-elbow prosthesis with a CAPP terminal device. For the past six months he has worn an M supracondylar below-elbow prosthesis with a Systemteknik (Swedish) hand and a UNB 1-site control system. The 1-site control system was selected because this child was unable to adequately isolate forearm flexor and extensor muscle group activity; the UNB system permits such co-contractions to be utilized for myoelectric control, whereas 2-site systems require alternating isolated flexor and extensor muscle activity. A myoelectrically-controlled toy train was used for the myoelectric testing and controls training during the initial five sessions; the child then received three sessions of prosthetic training to refine control and improve grasping patterns in all planes.

Although this child has found the myoelectric system to be heavier and to require more concentration to operate, he prefers the M device to his previous BP system, as do his parents and teacher. However, he has found speed of operation and appearance to be better with the CAPP terminal device. This is an exceptionally bright boy who perseveres and has much patience! No maintenance problems have been encountered with the hand, but gloves need to be replaced every two and a half months.

The second case, a seven year-old boy with a traumatic elbow disarticulation, was originally fitted with a BP prosthesis containing an external-locking elbow component and a voluntary opening (v.o.) hook terminal device. For the past nine months he has worn the Otto Bock myoelectric hand and continued to use the BP elbow unit.

Comfort of socket fit was satisfactory with both prostheses; he found the hand to be heavier but preferred the stronger grip it provided. He also preferred the appearance of the hand to that of the hook, and was observed using it with more spontaneity. The child grasped the concept of myoelectric control with ease, and controlled the device accurately. He felt that control was comparable to the hook. The child has been very active and not cautious about protecting the glove from soilage and tears. No maintenance problems have been encountered, however, save those related to the glove.

SUMMARY

The literature and our clinical experience indicate that there are both advantages and disadvantages to myoelectric prosthetic systems. While body-powered systems with hook terminal devices are perceived by users to be lighter-weight and maintenance-free, M systems with hand terminal devices are thought to be better looking and to permit more freedom of movement due to the absence of the control harness. No direct, empirical comparisons of myoelectric and body-powered hands are found in the literature.

TABLE 4-1. Terminal Devices and Prosthetic Systems Available for Two to Seven Year-Old Below-Elbow Amputees

A. TERMINAL DEVICES

Mechanical Hooks:
1. Hosmer/Dorrance Hooks; voluntary opening (v.o.)
   12P (for age range of 1 to 4)   2¾″ long; 1¾″ opening
   10P & 10X (for age range of 3 to 6)   3¼″ long; 2⅝″ opening
   99X (for age range of 6 to 10)   3¾″ long; 3½″ opening
2. CAPP Terminal Device; for children up to age 7; 2¹⁵⁄₁₆″ long; v.o.; center pull
3. TRS A.D.E.P.T. terminal device; voluntary closing (v.c.) (aluminum with polymer covering)

Mechanical Hands:
1. Dorrance v.o. size 6½-7   Actually designed for child age 8 to 10.
2. Otto Bock v.o. 6¾   A 7 year old could conceivably use this t.d.
3. Variety Village (model 102)-cable operated to activate the thumb. Only provides lateral key pinch; fingers are fixed in a partially flexed position; (for age 4 to 7; 2 lb. pinch

Powered Hands:
1. Systemteknik Myoelectric Hand (age 2 to 6½); Swedish Hand-2″ opening
2. Steeper Myoelectric Hand (6 to 8 year old); resembles Swedish Hand (English)-2¼″ opening
3. Otto Bock 8E14 (8 to 12 year old); 2⅜″ opening.
4. Variety Village (model 105; 3 to 6 year old) and (model 106; 3 to 10 year old); myoelectric or switch controlled; resembles Swedish Hand-model 105; 1½″ opening; model 106; 2.2″ opening; 3 to 5 lbs. grasp for both models.

B. CONTROL SYSTEMS
1. Body Powered Controlled Prostheses; Sockets and Control Systems
   a. Standard BE with figure "8" harness
   b. Muenster (Hepp-Kuhn)-cast in 90° for very short below elbow; figure 9 harness
   c. Supracondylar (for short residuum cast in 20°-90°, for long residuum cast 45°; figure 9 harness; (Northwestern design)
      Pressure high over the epicondyles and allows for lower anterior trim to decrease restriction to elbow flexion; figure 9 used harness for cable control.
   d. Pre-flexed socket (flex of 20°-25° of forearm section; "banana" shaped); figure "8" harness
   e. Split-socket for increased elbow flexion range and figure "8" harness
2. Myoelectric Prosthesis
   Sockets (BE)
   a. Muenster socket
   b. Supracondylar design
   Control Systems
   a. Otto Bock   3 state (1 site) or 2 state (2 sites) systems
   b. UNB   3 state (1 site) system

Table 4-2. Functional Comparison of Terminal Devices and Prosthetic Systems Available for Two to Seven Year-Old Below-Elbow Amputees

I. Prehension Factors:

Hooks	CAPP	Hands (mechanical and myoelectric)
1) offers precision prehension	offers coarse prehension	offers coarse 3 point prehension
2) finger moves in a transverse/ horizontal plane	movement of operating lever on a sagittal/ vertical plane—with center pull	movement of the thumb and first two fingers in a sagittal/vertical plane
3) grasping objects from table top level usually accomplished with ease	grasp of small objects from table top awkward and at times not possible; operating level must be turned toward midline to have object in view & child may have to stand	grasp of small objects from table top awkward or not possible; compensatory motions of arm abduction and internal rotation with/ without standing
4) visibility of objects good in all positions	visibility best in or toward mid position and in supination	visibility best in mid position and supination—more surface occluded by hand
5) for more stability, objects can be positioned diagonally across thumb post	objects positioned at right angle to operating lever for more surface to contact friction pad for good stability	larger contoured (round) objects which offer more surface contact are grasped with stability
6) good use in "hooking" mode ie: good for climbing on playground equipment	not good for hooking mode	partially useful for "hooking"—need to open hand to grasp
7) weight satisfactory	weight satisfactory	heavy
8) t.d. can be opened with ease as compared with other t.d.'s—prehension force is controlled by number of tension bands applied; equivalent of 1 lb. per full band (approx.)	more difficult to activate than hook but less than hand; prehension force limited; to achieve 1½ lb. pinch requires 5 to 6 lb. pull (approx.)	mechanical hand requires more energy expenditure to activate; myoelectric hand requires more concentration to activate; good grip strength; range from 3 lbs. to 13 lbs.

Table 4-2. *(Continued)*

I. Prehension Factors:

Hooks	CAPP	Hands (mechanical and myoelectric)
9) span of opening: from 1¾″ to 3½″	span of opening: 2¾″	span of opening: from 1½″ to 2⅜″
10) plastisole covered—needs replacement periodically	cover needs to be replaced periodically	gloves need to be replaced frequently—average of 1 every 2-3 months for an active child

II. Prosthetic Actuation Factors:

	Myoelectric	Body Powered
Control in Space	a) self suspending with no harness (supracondylar and Muenster)	a) cable controlled with harness
	b) allows for unrestricted movement in space (behind head, above head, back & at floor level) with good control of the t.d. with fluid motion	b) t.d. opening behind head, above head and behind back is limited or not possible due to slack on cable; motions are more awkward to activate t.d. and require more effort—biscapular abduction needed to activate t.d. close to midline
	c) socket design restricts full elbow flexion and extension and more difficult to don and remove	
Comfort	a) weight—heavier due to hand & suspension than body powered	a) weight—lighter in weight with hook as t.d.
	b) instability of socket under load particularly in extension	b) more stability with figure "8" harness

42

Table 4-2. *(Continued)*

II. Prosthetic Actuation Factors:

	Myoelectric	Body Powered
Maintenance	repairs are more frequent than for body powered—most common: glove replacement, battery replacement	repairs are minor—harness, replacement of plastisol covering or CAPP cover
Function	overall function less—due to qualities of the hand (ie: no fine pinch, poorer visibility)	overall function better using hook than BP hand
Speed of Operation	speed of t.d. activation slower as compared with body powered; motivation may be greater to use myoelectric prosthesis despite the obvious functional disadvantages	speed faster than myoelectric but slower than sound hand

Chapter 5

David E. Krebs, PhD, PT

CONCLUSIONS AND FUTURE CONSIDERATIONS

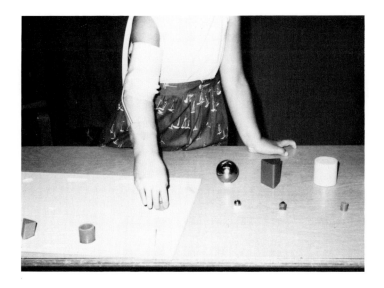

The assessment batteries for two to seven year-old unilateral below-elbow amputees which came out of the Symposium are listed in Appendix C; the Data Collection Form is shown in Appendix D. Although the Symposium was only a first step in the development of reliable and valid instruments to be used in functional assessment of pediatric upper-limb amputees, it seems clear that the participants accomplished their goal of inaugurating assessment batteries for pre-school children. The batteries must now be systematically and empirically evaluated to determine if they can indeed serve as valid prehension assessment tools for the pediatric upper-limb deficient population.

Certainly all tests should be malleable. The assessment batteries developed by the Symposium participants are provided as a starting point for the particular testing needs of the therapist who works with pre-school unilateral amputees; the tests may be made more useful if adapted specifically to the conceptual interests of a given tester. For example, if one wanted to determine timed normative values for pediatric prehension function, the activities might be modified to minimize cross-cultural and socioeconomic influences on the resulting values. If above-elbow or partial-hand amputee prehension assessments were to be conducted, the test batteries might be adapted to explore more precisely the characteristics of each prosthetic type and level of disability.

Finally, it should be noted that publication of the assessment batteries or the scoring methods in this book does not indicate test hegemony. Although standardized testing methods and task duration (timing) scoring methods are emphasized, it should be understood that qualitative assessment methods (such as rating the aesthetics, spontaneity, or skill of prosthesis use) can also be valuable in answering questions about the relative merits of various prosthetic treatments and other elements in rehabilitation of the upper-limb deficient child. Furthermore, no attempt has been made to delineate subjective reactions (such as comfort or appearance), or to develop a psychological assessment battery. These factors are of course critical to amputee rehabilitation, and are an important part of comprehensive assessments, but the Symposium considered only functional performance assessment.

47

In conclusion, the participants of the Symposium hope that these beginning efforts will be further developed and subjected to stringent tests of scientific merit, so that our knowledge of upper-limb prosthetic treatment options can keep pace with technological developments in the field.

APPENDICES

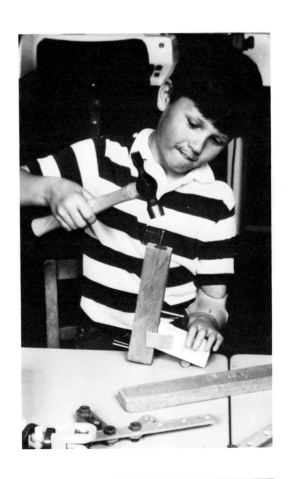

APPENDIX A

BIMANUAL PREHENSION TASKS FOR TWO TO SEVEN YEAR-OLD UNILATERAL BELOW-ELBOW AMPUTEES

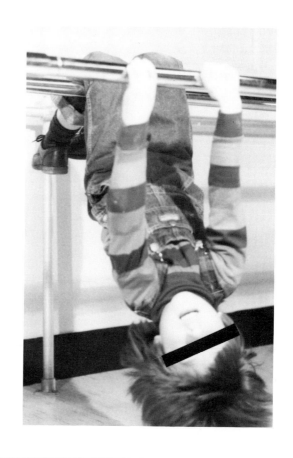

Each participant invited to the Symposium was asked to contribute tasks from the literature or clinical experience that she or he found useful in the treatment of unilateral upper-limb amputees. This task list provided the Symposium's participants with an initial pool of items that could be modified and thus fashioned into a prosthetic prehension test. These tasks were to be bimanual (because unilateral amputees will use the sound side to perform one-handed activities) and repetitive (to permit accurate performance testing). Thus, the following task list is presented in the spirit of historical accuracy for those interested in the origins of the prehension test, and also in the spirit of providing creative ideas for training pediatric unilateral below-elbow amputees in play, Activities of Daily Living, and other purposeful activities.

The tasks are arranged by increasing difficulty (approximately according to chronological age or developmental order) as judged by the Symposium participants. However, the items have not been empirically validated, so some may be quite inappropriate with respect to the age at which the amputee should be expected to perform the task. Furthermore, the manner in which a task is performed contributes to variability in performance results, and may in some cases invalidate the age ranges provided. Such disclaimers aside, however, at least some of the following items should be useful additions to the treatment armamentarium for the clinician and the researcher to build upon.

TASK	AGE (EST.)
Ride ride-on (tricycle)	1½-2½
Pull apart toys: e.g., Pop-It beads	2
String large objects: large beads, spool	2
Remove a toy from cloth drawstring bag: e.g., bubble gum bag	2
Don/doff mitt to sound hand, fasten Velcro at wrist	2
Open zippered pencil case, remove large felt pen, draw	2
Remove loose clothing: e.g., wool sweater/jumper from a doll	2
Open packages of cereal or raisins	2
Wind-up spring-propelled toys	2-2½
Open and close felt-tipped pens	2
Screw/unscrew nested Kittie-in-the-Kegs	3
Take off and put on prosthesis	3
Remove hard candy from wrapper	3
Wrap charm or little toy	3
Screw threaded rod-and-nut set	3
Blow soap bubbles	3
Grasp and pull up trousers or skirt	3
Grasp trousers and pull belt through loops, buckle	3
Remove and open facial tissue from purse-size package	3
Fill cup with water from low spigot	3
Remove soft (e.g., Kit-Kat) candy wrapper	3
"Shopping": push baby cart and pick up items from floor	3
Dry dishes	3
Open package of potato chips	3
Open and dump contents of 2 inch (restaurant-size) sugar package	4
Cut or tear 8 × 11 paper into quarters	4
Buckle belt mounted on table	4
Open and remove padlock	4
Peel a banana (started by therapist if necessary)	4
Sharpen pencil with hand-held sharpener	4
Grasp small orange and peel	4
Open toothpaste and apply to toothbrush	4
Sewing cards	4
Small bead stringing (macrame)	4-5
Hammer nails into wood	4-5
Apply bandaid to doll arm	4-5
Start and zip zipper	4-5
Cut 6 inch circle from 8 × 11 paper, paste to another paper	4-5
Unwrap a stick of gum	4-7

TASK	AGE (EST.)
Put curtains on rod	5
Sweep with brush and dust pan	5
Start and zip zipper of a jacket	5
Cut 6 inch circle from marked 8 × 11 paper	5
Tear many pieces of masking tape off roll	5
Grasp milk container and open	5
Tie a bow with large laces (boot provided) or lace boot on own foot	5-6
Fold paper, insert, and seal envelope	5-7
Shell a hardboiled egg	6
Grasp and pull on overshoes	6
Shuffle and deal 5 cards	7
Erector sets, meccanno	7
Use safety pin	7
Open a pat of jelly, spread butter on crackers	7
Roll paper and put rubber band around it	7
Leather work-lacing	7-8
Cut (hotdog or clay) meat with knife and fork	7-8
Sew on a button: cut length of thread (cotton) from spool (reel), thread needle, attach button to shirt	7-12
Wrap and tie package	5-7

APPENDIX B

GENERAL INSTRUCTIONS FOR TEST ADMINISTRATION

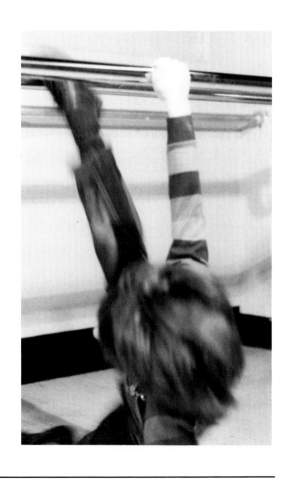

The purpose of the Pediatric Prehension Assessment is to provide a standard clinical assessment of pediatric below-elbow amputee function by objectively scoring Activities of Daily Living that compel repetitive terminal device (TD) use. If the results are to reflect TD skill accurately, testing error must be minimized, so the instructions should be followed rigorously.

AGE CATEGORY

Three separate test batteries have been constructed. These test batteries are denoted I, II, and III, and correspond roughly to the age groups of two to three, four to five, and six to seven respectively. For the assessment to accurately reflect all the domains tested by a given battery, the child must be able to complete all the tasks in that battery. If, for example, a four year-old is unable to perform all tasks from test battery II, test battery I should be utilized.

Please be sure to complete all the questions on the Data Collection Form and circle the test category used. If the child cannot complete all tasks in a given age category, note those that cannot be completed.

EQUIPMENT REQUIRED

Each task requires slightly different equipment. Be certain to have available all necessary equipment prior to the test session.

TESTING PROCEDURES

Conduct the test in a room free of auditory and visual distractions. Use a table and chair sized to suit the participant. Demonstrate each task in its entirety according to the instructions in the protocol; use your hand corresponding to the participant's amputated side as if it were a terminal device. Note particularly any prepositioning required. After demonstrating, replenish the test equipment if necessary, and return the items to the starting

59

position specified in the protocol. Do not allow the participant to practice the tasks.

Read the instructions in the protocol to the participant verbatim, referring to the prosthesis, terminal device, and sound hand by terms familiar to the participant. You may elaborate on the instructions **prior** to starting the test to remind the participant of the proper procedures. If the participant uses the terminal device only for stabilization, or stabilizes the prosthesis with the sound hand, remind him or her of the correct procedures by rereading instructions verbatim. Make no other comments during the testing. Be especially conscious not to "cheer" or encourage the participant during testing.

In general, younger children require more diversion time between tasks, and require some sort of reward for successfully completing the task. Choose a favorite play activity and permit the child to play and rest as much as necessary between each task performance.

SCORING METHOD

Record the time between test "start" and "stop" for each task. You may also rate the quality or spontaneity of TD use on an "Excellent-Good-Average-Poor-Cannot Complete" scale if desired.

PROBLEMS

Describe any difficulties encountered during the test session, or any variance from the test protocol, in the "Comments" section of the Data Collection Form.

APPENDIX C

ASSESSMENT BATTERIES FOR TWO TO SEVEN YEAR-OLD UNILATERAL BELOW- ELBOW AMPUTEES

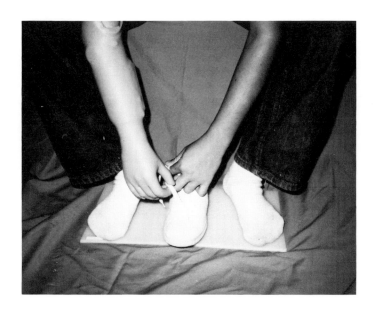

TASK	EQUIPMENT REQUIRED	POSITIONS
I.1. String 4 large beads	— 1″ Playskool beads: 1 Flat round 1 Cylinder 1 Ball 1 Hexagon — 12″ string knotted at one end, with 3″ reinforced tip. — Bowl.	— Child stands at table. — Therapist stands at amputated to demonstrate. — String on table on sound side 12″ anterior to elbow. — Beads in bowl on table, on prosthetic side, 12″ from table, directly in front of elbow.
I.2. Open 4 film cans	— 4 35mm film cans with flexible plastic lids secured; penny-sized item inside each.	— Child stands at table. — Therapist stands at amputated side to demonstrate. — Cans in therapist's pocket.
I.3. Separate 3 barrels	— Three nested screw-top barrels, closed snugly.	— Child stands at table. — Therapist stands at amputated side to demonstrate. — Barrels on table on prosthetic side, 12″ from table edge, directly in front of elbow.

INSTRUCTIONS	START/STOP
— Therapist demonstrates. — "Use your sound hand to place a bead in your terminal device. Grasp the string in your sound hand and lace the bead. Continue until you've strung all 4 beads."	Start: 1st bead touched. Stop: 4th bead strung. Maximum: 4 minutes.
— Therapist demonstrates. — "Grasp the can with your terminal device. Open the can, and remove the items. Put each opened can and item on the table." — Therapist gives 1 can at a time to the sound hand.	Start: 1st can held in sound hand. Stop: 4th lid placed on table.
— Therapist demonstrates. — "Open the barrels as fast as you can. Find what's inside."	Start: Barrels touched. Stop: Last barrel opened. Maximum: 4 minutes.

TASK	EQUIPMENT REQUIRED	POSITIONS
I.4. Assemble 10 interlocking beads	— 10 Magneto snap-beads, separated. — Bowl.	— Child sits at table. — Therapist sits at amputated side to demonstrate. — Beads in bowl on table on sound side, 12″ anterior to elbow.
I.5. Separate a 5 piece Lego bar	— 3 8-prong Lego bars. — 2 6-prong Lego bars.	— Child stands at table. — Therapist stands at amputated side to demonstrate. — Bars, assembled in a stack, on table on prosthetic side, 12″ from table edge, directly in front of elbow.

INSTRUCTIONS	START/STOP
— Therapist demonstrates. — "Take the beads, one at a time, from the bowl with your sound hand. Hold the beads in your T.D. while snapping them together. You'll need to re-grasp the chain near the end to attach the next one."	Start: 1st bead touched. Stop: 10th bead attached. Maximum: 4 minutes.
— Therapist demonstrates. — "Hold the Legos in your T.D. and pull them apart, one by one."	Start: Lego stack touched. Stop: 5th Lego separated. Maximum: 4 minutes.

TASK	EQUIPMENT REQUIRED	POSITIONS
II.1. Sew a sewing card	— Glossy finished, Fisher-Price bear or bunny sewing card. — Plastic lace with rigid tip.	— Child stands at table. — Therapist stands at amputated side to demonstrate. — Card on table on prosthetic side, 12″ from table edge, directly in front of elbow. — String on table on sound side, 12″ from table edge, directly in front of elbow. — TD fully supinated.
II.2. String 10 small beads	— 10½″ cube Milton-Bradley wooden beads. — 10″ string, knotted at one end, with ½″ reinforced tip. — Bowl.	— Child sits at table. — Therapist sits at amputated side to demonstrate. — String on table on sound side, 12″ anterior to elbow. — Beads in bowl on table on prosthetic side, 12″ anterior to elbow.
II.3. Stick a bandage to the table	— Curad "Ouchless" ¾″ plastic bandage in paper package.	— Child stands at table. — Therapist stands at amputated side to demonstrate. — Bandage on table on sound side, 12″ from table edge, directly in front of elbow.

INSTRUCTIONS	START/STOP
— Therapist demonstrates by lacing first 3 holes. — Card is to be removed from TD and turned over for each successive hole so that lace is always inserted *down* into hole *from above.* — "Grasp the card with your terminal device the same way I showed you. Turn the card over after every hole is sewn. Continue for 5 holes."	Start: Card grasped. Stop: 5th hole laced. Maximum: 4 minutes.
— Therapist demonstrates. — "Use your sound hand to place a bead in the terminal device. Grasp the string in your sound hand and lace the bead. Release the bead to string the next. Continue until you've strung all the beads."	Start: 1st bead grasped. Stop: 10th bead strung. Maximum: 6 minutes.
— Therapist demonstrates. — "Grasp the bandage tops with both hands. Pull the paper open. Remove both adhesive backs, then stick the bandage to the table."	Start: Bandage touched. Stop: Both tabs stuck to table. Maximum: 5 minutes.

TASK	EQUIPMENT REQUIRED	POSITIONS
II.4. Cut a paper circle and glue it to another paper. 	— 6″ circle drawn on construction paper, 8¼ ×10½″. — Blank sheet of 9×12″ construction paper. — Blunt scissors, left- or right-handed to suit sound side. — 1¼ oz. oval plastic bottle of white glue, *closed*.	— Child sits at table. — Therapist sits on amputated side to demonstrate. — Items arranged on table, as shown below.
II.5. Open package and remove tissues	— 2 "Purse-size" tissue packages, unopened.	— Child stands at table. — Therapist faces child. — Tissue package on table on prosthetic side 12″ anterior to elbow.

INSTRUCTIONS	START/STOP
— Therapist demonstrates, leaves completed papers on table for child's reference. — "Hold the paper in your terminal device. Cut along the line with the scissors held in your sound hand. Turn the paper whenever you need to. Hold the glue bottle in your terminal device to open it. Apply 6 drops of glue, and glue the circle to the other paper. Neatness counts."	Start: Paper grasped. Stop: Circle glued to blank paper. Circle must be cut within 1 inch of line. If not, repeat the task. Maximum: 7 minutes.
— Therapist demonstrates. — "Hold the package with your terminal device. Open it with your sound hand. Then take out 1 tissue, and put it on the table. Do the same thing with the second package."	Start: Package grasped. Stop: Tissue removed from second package. Maximum: 5 minutes.

TASK	EQUIPMENT REQUIRED	POSITIONS
III.1. Cut "meat"	— ½ can Play-Doh molded into round ½″ thick pattie, surface scored in 4 strips. — Plastic plate on wet paper towel to stabilize plate. — Bowl.	— Participant sits at table. — Therapist sits at amputated side to demonstrate; stands behind participant during test with hand near participant's mouth. — Items arranged on table:
III.2. Cut geometric shape 	— 20 lb. bond paper, 8½ ×11″ in the center of which appears a 6″ circle with 90° wedge design — Blunt scissors, left- or right-handed to suit sound side.	— Participant stands at table. — Therapist stands at amputated side to demonstrate. — Paper on table on amputated side, 12″ from table edge. — Scissors on table on sound side, 12″ from table edge.

70

INSTRUCTIONS	START/STOP
— Therapist demonstrates — "Put the fork in your terminal device. Stab the meat with the fork. Cut along the mark with the knife held in your sound hand. *Switch the fork to your sound hand* to remove the piece from the plate and give it to me as if you were going to eat it. Put the fork back in your terminal device to cut the next piece. Continue until you have given me all 4 pieces." — Therapist takes each piece from fork then puts piece in bowl.	Start: Fork touched. Stop: 4th piece given to therapist. Maximum: 4 minutes.
— Therapist demonstrates. — "Hold the paper in your terminal device. Do not allow the paper to touch the table. Cut along the line with the scissors held in your sound hand. Turn the paper whenever you need to. Neatness counts."	Start: Paper touched. Stop: Design cut completely. Shape must have 70-110° angle, and be cut within ½" of line. If not, repeat the task. Maximum: 6 minutes.

TASK	EQUIPMENT REQUIRED	POSITIONS
III.3. Discard 5 red playing cards	— 10 playing cards stacked so that red and black cards alternate	— Participant sits at table. — Therapist sits at amputated side to demonstrate. — Cards stacked on table on sound side, 12″ anterior to elbow.
III.4. Lace top four holes of shoe or boot, and tie a single bow.	— Child's own shoe is preferred, on foot of child's choice. Four holes unlaced. — Have large-sized lace shoe available, with reinforced tip cotton laces.	— Child on floor, limb position is his/her own choice. — Therapist sits at amputated side to demonstrate.
III.5. Wrap book	— Paperback book, about 7 ½ × 4½ × ½″ — Cellophane tape in light weight dispenser — 20 lb. bond paper, 8½ ×11″	— Participant stands at table. — Therapist stands at amputated side to demonstrate. — Tape dispenser placed over book which lies atop paper on table 12″ directly in front of participant.

INSTRUCTIONS	START/STOP
— Therapist demonstrates. — "Hold the cards in your terminal device so you can see them all. Discard the 5 red cards, one at a time. Be careful not to drop any cards."	Start: Cards touched. Stop: 5th card discarded. Maximum: 3 minutes.
— Therapist demonstrates. — "Lace the shoe and tie the bow as you usually do. Be sure it is tight."	Start: 1st lace touched. Stop: Bow completed. Maximum: 5 minutes.
— Therapist demonstrates. — "Wrap the book so it is all covered. Put 1 piece of tape on the back and 2 pieces at each end. Neatness does not count."	Start: Tape dispenser touched. Stop: 5th tape applied. Maximum: 6 minutes.

73

APPENDIX D

DATA COLLECTION FORM

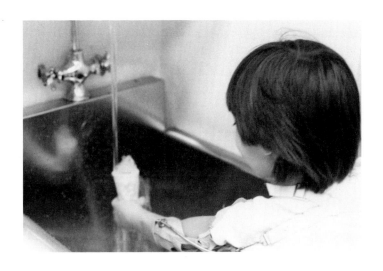

Prehension Assessment for Unilateral Below-Elbow Amputees

Tester Name _____ Clinic Name _____ Today's Date ___/___/___

Child Name _____ Date of Birth ___/___/___ Height _____ Weight _____ Sex _____

Amputation Date ___/___/___ Amputation Type _____ Stump Length (epicondyle to distal end) _____

Age at first prosthetic fitting: Passive _____ Active _____ Prosthetic use: Hrs/Day _____ Days/Wk _____

Current Components (give catalogue number where possible): Terminal Device(s) _____

Wrist _____ Control System _____ Socket Type _____ Harness Type _____

Number and duration of therapy sessions with current prosthesis _____

Circle test category performed: I   II   III   Can child perform all items in this category? _____

TEST RESULTS

Task Number	Trial 1 Score	Trial 2 Score	Comments

BIBLIOGRAPHY

Agnew, P.J., Shannon, G.F.: Training Program for a Myoelectrically Controlled Prosthesis with Sensory Feedback System. Am. J. Occ. Ther. 35:722-727, 1981.

American Guidance Service Inc.: Minnesota Rate of Manipulation Test: The Placing Test. Circle Pines, MN: American Guidance Service Inc., 1969.

Ames, L.B. et al.: The Gesell Institute's Child from One to Six: Evaluating the Behaviour of the Preschool Child. New York: Harper and Row, 1979.

Anderson, M., Sollars, R., Winston, M.: Manual of Arm Amputee Checkout and Training. Los Angeles: UCLA School of Medicine, Prosthetics Education Program, 1957.

Angliss,V.E.: Habilitation of Upper Limb Deficient Children. Am. J. Occ. Ther. 28:407-414, 1974.

Ayres, A.J.: Sensory Integration and Learning Disorders. Los Angeles: Western Psychological Services, 1972. pp. 248-255.

Baron, E., Clark, S.D., Solomon, C.: The Two Stage Myoelectric Hand for Children and Young Adults. Ortho and Pros. 37(2):11-24, 1983.

Bayley, N.: The Development of Motor Abilities During the First Three Years: Monographs of the Society for Research in Child Development. No. 1. Washington DC: Society for Research in Child Development National Research Council, 1935.

Bergholtz, S.G.: Evaluation of the Area Child Amputee Clinic (ACAC) Electric Hook. New York: Prosthetics and Orthotics, New York University Post-Graduate Medical School, 1976.

Blakeslee, B.: The Limb-Deficient Child. Berkeley, CA: University of California Press, 1963.

Brooks, M., Shaperman, J.: Infant Prosthetic Fitting: A Study of the Results. Am. J. Occ. Ther. 29:329-334, 1965.

Caplan, F., Caplan, T.: The Power of Play. Garden City, NY: Doubleday, 1973.

_____: The Second Twelve Months of Life. New York: Bantam, 1977.

CAPP: First Annual Report. Los Angeles: UCLA Department of Engineering, 1955.

_____: Second Annual Report. Los Angeles: UCLA Department of Pediatrics, School of Medicine, 1956.

_____: Third Annual Report. Los Angeles: UCLA Department of Pediatrics, School of Medicine, 1957.

_____: Seventh Annual Report. Los Angeles: UCLA Department of Pediatrics, School of Medicine, 1961.

Carroll, D.: A Quantitative Test of Upper Extremity Function. J. Chron. Dis. 18:479-491, 1965.

Challenor, Y., Rangaswany, L., Katz, J.: Limb Deficiency in Infancy and Childhood. In Downey J., Low, N.: The Child with a Disabling Illness: Principles of Rehabilitation. New York: Haven Press, 1982.

Clarke, S.D.: Delivery of Occupational Therapy Services for the Child Amputee: Optimum Procedures and Problems. In Proceedings, Symp. Child Amp. Mgmnt. Atlanta, 1973.

_____: A Developmental Approach to Treatment Planning for the Limb Deficient Child. In Proceedings, 8th Int. Cong. World Fed. Occ. Ther. Hamburg, West Germany, 1982.

Clarke, S.D., Patton, J.G.: Occupational Therapy for the Limb Deficient Child. Clin. Orthop. and Rel. Res. 148:47-50, 1980.

Coley, I.: Pediatric Assessment of Self-Care Activities. St. Louis: Mosby, 1978.

Davies, E., Fritz, B., Clippinger, F.: Children with Amputations. Inter-Clinic Inform. Bull. 9:19-48, 1969.

Day, H.J.B.: The United Kingdom Trial of the Swedish Myoelectric Hand for Young Children: An Interim Report. Inter-Clinic Inform. Bull. 17(8):5-8, 1980.

Denckla, M.B.: Development of Motor Co-ordination in Normal Children. Develop. Med. Child Neurol. 16:729-741, 1974.

Dennis, J.F.: Infant and Child Upper Extremity Amputees: Their Prosthesis and Training. J. Rehab. 28(2):26-28, 1962.

Durance, F.P., O'Shea, B.J.: An Evaluation of Upper Limb Amputees. Kingston, Ontario: Internal Report, Regional Rehabilitation Centre, Kingston General Hospital, September 1981.

Erhardt, R.P.: Sequential Levels in Development of Prehension. Am. J. Occ. Ther. 28:592-596, 1975.

_____: Developmental Hand Dysfunction: Theory, Assessment and Treatment. Laurel, MD: RAMSCO, 1982.

Fisher, A.G.: Initial Prosthetic Fitting of the Congenital Below-Elbow Amputee: Are we Fitting them Early Enough? Inter-Clinic Inform. Bull. (11&12):7-10, 1976.

Fishman, S.: Behavioral and Psychological Reactions of Juvenile Amputees. In Swinyard C (ed.): Limb Development and Deformity -- Problems of Evaluation and Rehabilitation, Chapter Eight. Springfield, IL: Charles Thomas, 1969.

81

Fishman, S., Kay, H.W.: Acceptability of a Functional-Cosmetic Artificial Hand for Young Children, Part 1. Artif. Limbs 8(1)28-43, 1964.

_____: Acceptability of a Functional-Cosmetic Artificial Hand for Young Children, Part 2. Artif. Limbs 8(2): 15-27, 1964.

Fletcher, M.J., Leonard, F.: The Principles of Artifical-Hand Design. Artific. Limbs 2(2):78-94, 1955.

Florey, L.: An Approach to Play and Play Development. Am. J. Occ. Ther. 25(6):275-280, 1971.

Ford, E.R. et al.: Studies of the Upper Extremity Amputee. Artif. Limbs 5(2):4-128, 1958.

Fraiberg, S.: The Magic Years. New York: Scribner, 1959.

Franz, C.: A New Venture. Inter-Clinic Inform. Bull. 1(1):1, 1961.

_____: Evolution in the Care of the Child Amputee. Artific. Limbs 10(1):2-4, 1966.

French, R.W.: Motor Development and Intellectual Functioning: An Exploratory Study. Inter-Clinic Inform. Bull. 12(8):13-15, 1973.

Gesell, A. et al.: The First Five Years of Life. New York: Harper and Row, 1940.

Gesell, A., Amatruda, C.S.: Developmental Diagnosis: Normal and Abnormal Child Development. New York: Paul B. Hoeber Inc., 1941.

Gilad, I.: Motion Pattern Analysis for Evaluation and Design of a Prosthetic Hook. Arch. Phys. Ed. Rehabil. 66:399-401, 1985.

Gilfoyle, E.M., Grady, A.P., Moore, J.C.: Children Adapt. Thorofare, NJ: Slack, 1981.

Gortons A.: Field Study -- Dorrance Model 2 Hand. Technical Report. New York: Prosthetic and Orthotics, New York University Post-Graduate Medical School, 1967.

Herberts, P. et al.: Rehabilitation of Unilateral Below Elbow Amputees with Myoelectric Prostheses. Scand. J. Rehab. Med. 12:123-128, 1980.

Hopkins, H., Smith, H.: Willard and Spackman's Occupational Therapy. (ed. 5). Philadelphia: Lippincott and Co., 1978.

Hubbard, S.: The Development of the Myoelectric Training Methods for Pre-School Congenital Below-Elbow Amputees and the Comparison of Two Training Protocols. Ontario Crippled Children's Center, Technical Report. Ontario, 1983.

Illingworth, R.S.: The Development of the Infant and Young Child: Normal and Abnormal. (ed. 6). London: Churchill Livingstone, 1975.

Ingvarsson, B. et al.: Proposal for Test Instructions for Clinical Testing of Prostheses for Unilateral Upper Limb Amputees. Linkoping, Sweden: Lab. Rehab. Eng., Dept. Rehab. Med., University Hospital, 1980.

Jebsen, R.H. et al.: Objective and Standardized Test of Hand Function. Arch. Phys. Med. Rehabil. 50:311-319, 1969.

Kay, H.W., Peizer, E.: Studies of the Upper-Extremity Amputee. VI. Prosthetic Usefulness and Wearer Performance. Artific. Limbs 5(2):31-87, 1958.

Keith, R.A.: Functional Assessment Measures in Medical Rehabilitation, Current Status. Arch. Phys. Med. Rehabil. 65:74-78, 1984.

Kellor, M., Frost, J., Silberberg, N.: Hand Strength and Dexterity. Am. J. Occup. Ther. 25:77-83, 1971.

Kopp, C.B., Shaperman, J.: Cognitive Development in the Absence of Object Manipulation During Infancy. Develop. Psychol. 9(3):1973.

Krebs, D., Fishman, S.: Characteristics of the Child Amputee Population. J. Ped. Orthop. 4:89-95, 1984.

Lamb, D.W., Scott, H.: Management of Congenital and Acquired Amputation in Children. Orthop. Clin. N. Amer. 12(4):977-994, 1981.

Lambert, C., Sciora, J.: Questionnaire of Juvenile to Young Adult Amputees Who Have Had Prostheses Supplied to Them Through the University of Illnois Division of Services for Crippled Children. J. Bone Joint Surg. 41A:1437-1454, 1959.

Law, H.T.: Engineering of Upper Limb Prostheses. Orthop. Clin. N. Am. 12:929-951, 1981.

Lehneis, H.R.: Methods-Time Measurement as a Basis of Evaluation of Performance of Standardized Tasks of Upper Limb Amputees with Conventional and Myo-electrically-Controlled Prostheses. PhD Dissertation, New York University, 1975.

Lund, A.: Observations on the Very Young Upper Extremity Amputee. Am. J. Occ. Ther. 12:15-36, 1958.

MacDonald, R.: Occupational Therapy in Rehabilitation. (ed. 3). London, England: Baillierre, Tindall and Cassell, 1970.

MacDonell, J.A.: Age of Fitting Upper-Extremity Prostheses in Children: A Clinical Study. J. Bone and Joint Surg. 40A:655-662, 1958.

Maier, H.W.: Three Theories of Child Development: New York: Harper and Row, 1965.

McWilliam, R.P.J.G.: A List of Everyday Tasks for Use in Prosthesis Design and Development. Bull. Pros. Res. 10-13:135-164, 1970.

Mendez, A.M.: A Trial to Evaluate a Myoelectric Prosthesis for Young Children with a Single Below Elbow Absence. In Proceedings, 8th Int. Cong. World Fed. Occ. Ther. Hamburg, West Germany, 1982.

Michigan Area Child Amputee Program. Training Program (syllabus and course notes by Julie Shaperman), 1957.

Millstein, S., Heger, H., Hunter, G.L: A Review of the Failures in Use of the Below Elbow Myoelectric Prosthesis. Orth. and Pros. 36(2):29-34, 1982.

New York University Post-Graduate Medical School: Prosthetics and Orthotics: Studies of the Upper Extremity Amputee. Artific. Limbs 5(1):4-94, 1958.

_____: Prosthetics and Orthotics: Upper Limb Prosthetics (Revision). New York: New York University Post-Graduate Medical School, 1982.

Noller, K., Ingrisano, D.: Cross-Sectional Study of Gross and Fine Motor Development: Birth to 6 Years of Age. Phys. Ther. 64:308-316, 1984.

Northmore-Ball, M.D., Heger, H., Hunter, G.A.: The Below-Elbow Myoelectric Prosthesis: A Comparison of the Otto Bock Myoelectric Prosthesis with the Hook and Functional Hand. J. Bone Joint Surg. 62B:363-367, 1980.

O'Shea, B.J.: Upper Limb Amputees: Functional Evaluation. In Proceedings, 1st Can. Cong. Rehabil. Ottowa, Canada, 1983.

O'Shea, B.J., Dunfield, V.A.: Myoelectric Training for Preschool Children. Arch. Phys. Med. Rehabil. 64: 451-455, 1983.

Paciga, J.E. et al.: Clinical Evaluation of UNB 3-State Myoelectric Control for Arm Prostheses. Bull. Pros. Res. 10-34:21-33, 1980.

Patton, J., Clarke, S.: Occupational Therapy for the Limb-Deficient Child: A Developmental Approach to Treatment and Planning and Selection of Prostheses for Infants and Young Children with Unilateral Upper Extremity Limb Deficiencies. Clin. Orthop. and Rel. Res. 148:47-54, 1980.

Peizer, E. et al.: Studies of the Upper Extremity Amputee. Artif. Limbs 5(1):4-94, 1958.

PEPAC Workshop in Prosthetics and Orthotics for Faculty Members in Schools of Occupational and Physical Therapy: Final Evaluation Report. Washington, DC: Vocational Rehabilitation Administration, 1965.

Pillet, J.: The Aesthetic Hand Prosthesis. Orthop. Clin. N. Am. 12:961-969, 1981.

Prosthetic-Orthotic Education: Management of the Juvenile Amputee. Evanston, IL: Northwestern University Medical School, 1963.

Pulaski, M.A.S.: Your Baby's Mind and How It Grows: Piaget's Theory for Parents. New York: Harper and Row, 1978.

Richardson, G., Lund, A.: Upper Extremity Prosthetic Training for the Young Amputee. Am. J. Occ. Ther. 13:15-63, 1959.

Robertson, E.: Rehabilitation of Arm Amputees and Limb Deficient Children. London, England: Baillierre, Tindall and Cassell, 1978.

Rodgers, C.D., Scott, R.N.: Early Fitting of Congenital Amputees with Powered Prostheses. Research Report 80-1. Fredericton, New Brunswick: Bio-Engineering Institute, University of New Brunswick, 1980.

Santschi, W.: Manual of Upper Extremity Prosthetics. Los Angeles: UCLA Department of Engineering, 1958.

Schultz, C.F., Kritter, A.E.: Myoelectric Single-Site Electrode Fitting for a Short Below-Elbow Amputee. Inter-Clinic Inform. Bull. 28(3):1-6, 1983.

Scott, R.N. (ed.): Myoelectric Prostheses for Very Young Children. Technical Report 82-1. Fredericton, New Brunswick: University of New Brunswick, 1981.

Setoguchi, Y., Rosenfelder, R.: The Limb Deficient Child. Springfield, IL: Charles Thomas, 1982.

Shaperman, J.: The Child Amputee: Observations on the Sequence of Learning Active Terminal Device Control. MA Thesis, University of Southern California, Los Angeles, 1960.

_____: Orientation to Prosthesis Use for the Child Amputee. Am. J. Occ. Ther. 14:17-26, 1960.

_____: Learning Techniques Applied to Prehension. Am. J. Occ. Ther. 14:70-74, 1960.

_____: A Comparison of Two Infant Terminal Devices. Inter-Clinic Inform. Bull. 3(1):1-6, 1964.

_____: Early Learning of Hook Operation. Inter-Clinic Inform. Bull. 14(9&10):11-18, 1975.

_____: Learning Patterns of Young Children with Above-Elbow Prostheses. Am. J. Occ. Ther. 33:299-305, 1979.

_____: Hands On: Prosthetics. Phys. Disabil. Section Newsletter, AOTA, 2(4):1-4, 1979.

Shaperman, J., Brooks, M.B., Campbell, H.E.: Developmental Factors in Infant Upper Extremity Prosthesis Fitting. Orthop. Pros. Appliance J. 15(2):148-158, 1961.

Sharples, N.: Child Amputees: Disability Outcomes and Antecedents. Final Report, July 1969 Initial Follow-Up Study of Selected Patients of an In-Patient Service. Ann Arbor, MI: University of Michigan, School of Public Health, 1969.

Sheridan, M.A.: Children's Developmental Progress: From Birth to Five Years (ed. 3). Atlantic Highlands, NJ: Humanities Press Inc., 1975.

Smith, H.B.: Smith Hand Function Evaluation. Am. J. Occ. Ther. 27(5):244-251, 1973.

Sorbye, R.: Myoelectric Controlled Hand Prostheses in Children. Int. J. Rehab. Res. 1:15-25, 1977.

_____: Myoelectric Prosthetic Fitting in Young Children. Clin. Orthop. Rel. Res. 148:34-40, 1980.

Stein, R.B., Walley, M.: Functional Comparison of Upper Extremity Amputees Using Myoelectric and Conventional Prostheses. Arch. Phys. Med. Rehabil. 64:243-248, 1983.

Strong, F.: Artificial Limbs -- Today and Tomorrow. Artif. Limbs 1(1):1-3, 1954.

Sypniewksi, B.: The Child with Terminal Transverse Partial Hemimelia: A Review of the Literature on Prosthetic Management. Artif. Limbs 16(1):29-50, 1972.

Teska, A., Swinyard, C.A.: Evaluation of a Standardized Test for Child's APRL-Sierra No. 1 Hand. Am. J. Occup. Ther. 15(1):17-18, 1961.

Trefler, E.: Let's Put a Hand on Captain Hook. Inter-Clinic Inform. Bull. 13(12):7-12, 1974.

Trost, F.J.: A Comparison of Conventional and Myoelectric Below-Elbow Prosthetic Use. Inter-Clinic Inform. Bull. 18(4):9-16, 1983.

Vulpe, S.: Vulpe Assessment Battery for the Atypical Child. Toronto: National Inst. on Mental Retard., 1978.

Warner, R.: A Philosophy and Technique of Child Amputee Management. Inter-Clinic Inform. Bull. 1(8):7-12, 1962.

Weiss-Lambrou, R.: A Manual for the Congenital Unilateral Below-Elbow Child Amputee. Am. Occ. Ther. Assoc: Rockville, MD, 1981.

Wellerson, T.: A Manual for Occupational Therapists on the Rehabilitation of the Upper Extremity Amputee. New York: American Occupational Therapy Association, 1958.

Wendt, J.D., Shaperman, J.: The Infant with a Cable-Controlled Hook: A Study of Development of Prehension Patterns. Am. J. Occ. Ther. 24:393-402, 1970.

Wilson, B.: Limb Prosthetics Today. Artif. Limbs 7(2):1-42, 1963.